Weight Loss Epiphany

The Workbook

Simple Strategies to Build Your Self Esteem and Release Weight

Angie J. Hernandez, C.Ht.

Disclaimer

The Publisher and the Author make no representations or warranties regarding the accuracy or completeness of the contents of this work and specifically disclaim all warranties, including without limitation, warranties of fitness for a particular purpose. No warranty may be created or extended by sales or promotional materials. The advice and strategies contained herein may not be suitable for every situation or person. This work is sold with the understanding that the Publisher is not engaged in rendering legal, accounting, medical, health or other professional services. If professional assistance is required, the services of a competent professional person should be sought. Neither the Publisher nor the Author shall be liable for damages arising here from. That an organization or website is referred to in this work as a citation and /or a potential source of further information does not mean that the Author or the Publisher endorse the information, the organization or website may provide or recommendations it may make. Further, readers should know that internet websites listed in this work may have changed or disappeared between when this work was written and when read. This is not medical advice. Always visit your doctor before starting any change in diet or exercise.

To Gamal, my biggest supporter.

Because you believed in me, I could believe in myself.

—Angie

TABLE OF CONTENTS

More Than Just A Book!

Free Video Sessions

Introduction to Weight Loss Epiphany

Week One

    1) Define Your Goal

    2) Create Your Own Goals

    3) Swiss Cheese Your Motivation

    4) Calculate Your Future Weight for an Upcoming Event

    5) Picture Yourself at Your Goal Weight

    6) Week One Homework

Week Two

    1) The Walking Challenge

    2) The Four Keys to Weight Loss Success

    3) Show off and hang your new piece of clothing

    4) Slim and Fit Thinking vs. Fat Thinking

    5) Week Two Homework

Week Three

    1) Re-cap Your Walking Challenge

    2) Write a Self Image Paragraph

    3) Learn Self-Hypnosis

    4) Week Three Homework

Week Four

1) Learn the Four R's

2) A Personal Injury Suit against Perfectionism

3) A Thank You Note

4) A Talk From Your Old Self

5) Your last homework assignment

MORE THAN JUST A BOOK!

Hypnosis

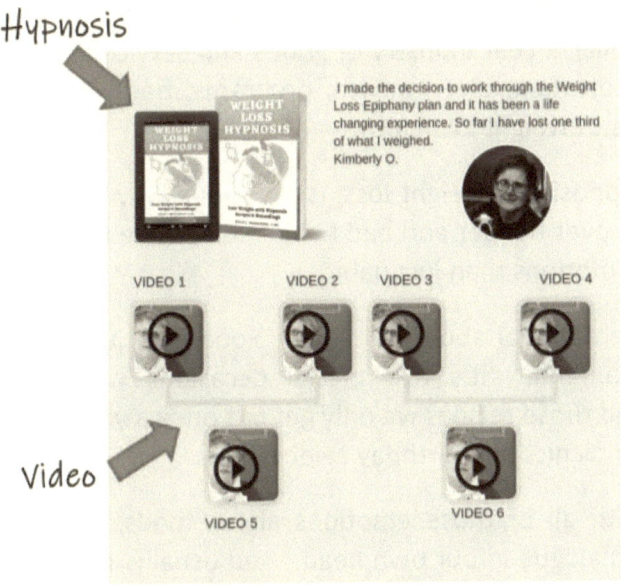

Video

FREE TRAINING: Video, Hypnosis

You have the book now get the step by step-step system I use for *in-person* Weight Loss Epiphany Clients with this link:

https://indianahypnosiscenter.com/wle-sessions/

I'll see you on the inside!

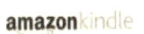   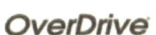

Introduction to Weight Loss Epiphany

Weight loss is not easy. If it were easy, there would not be a billion dollar a year industry of goods and services. We wouldn't need medication, diets, advice, programs, boot camps, exercise machines or weight loss clubs.

Using hypnosis for weight loss, is a positive way to give a person the edge over hunger and bad habits. But there is even more yet to food emotions than just habit.

We are emotional about our food. Food isn't just fuel, it's love from Grandma. It's the special occasions with friends and family and those recipes we only get out once a year. And it's pot lucks and picnics and birthday celebrations.

Along with all of those emotions about foods, we also have a running dialogue in our own head. And usually, that dialog is not too kind. That voice in our head berates us and puts us down and undermines the good work we do. Even when we eat well and are losing weight, it tells us that we are not good enough. That voice in our heads is a bully.

The Weight Loss Epiphany Workbook is designed to help squash the bully. We want to train the bully to be a supporter. Yes, it can be done! With the exercises outlined in the book, you are training that bully in your head, to change the way she talks to you. You are working at a new framework for inner speech that is supportive and loving. Combine that with the Hypnosis for Weight Loss and video training, and you have a winning combination!

XO,
Angie

Week One

You've embarked on a life change today and just by sitting down with this workbook, you're well into the first few steps of your journey. This is a program to lose weight or release weight as I like to say, but it's not only that.

This is also a journey of self-discovery. We don't just eat to fuel our bodies, we have emotional attachments to food. Learning more about ourselves while improving our health is a life bonus.

If you haven't joined the Facebook group yet, it's time to join now. We support one another and learn from one another there. Come on over!

In Week One, you will:

- Define Your Goal

- Create Your Own Goals

- Swiss Cheese Your Motivation

- Calculate your future weight for an upcoming event

- Picture yourself at your goal weight

- Receive your week one homework assignment.

1) Define Your Goal

You might wonder about the purpose of a written assignment, after all, you bought the program, isn't that enough to turn your bad habits around?

Your Subconscious Mind relates to the world through all of its senses; touch, sight, sound, smell, and taste. When you only engage part of the senses, you limit your chances of success.

In the Weight Loss Epiphany Program, you will be appealing to all five senses whenever possible. Those who find the most long-term success with this program, are those that embrace each part of it wholly.

Writing is an important part of success because handwriting is a learned response leading the information directly into your Subconscious Mind.

To define your goal, follow these guidelines:

1. Use only positive statements stated in the present tense. Eliminate words such as no, not, won't, don't, can't, try or want. When your Subconscious Mind hears a negative, it simply disregards it, making the rest of the thought even stronger.

Let's say you were on a diet where no cake was allowed but you LOVE chocolate cake. I'll bet you have been on a diet like that! So you tell yourself, "I will not eat chocolate cake, I do not want chocolate cake, I will not even think about chocolate cake!" But this is what your Subconscious Mind hears, "I will ~~not~~ eat chocolate cake, I do ~~not~~ want chocolate cake, I will ~~not~~ even think about chocolate cake!"

Whaaaat? Your Subconscious Mind crosses out the negative words and sees that chocolate cake is very important to you so it *HELPS* you by sending you thoughts of chocolate cake more often! Don't believe me? I'll prove it.

Don't think of a giant purple banana! Do not think of a giant purple banana. Don't even let a giant purple banana come into your head!

Of course, now, that's all you can think of. Giant purple bananas everywhere!

So, if you want to stop eating junky foods, avoid saying, "I want to stop eating junk food." Instead, state the positive way you'll be eating, "I eat fruits, vegetables and lean protein each day."

If you want to curb your portions, choose positive wording like, "I can feel satisfied with small, very filling amounts."

If you plan to exercise often, you might say it like this, "I take recess three times a week and I love it!"

In Your Notebook:

Write three positive statements about your weight release outcome.

1) Write this one about your exercise level. You may want to increase it or try something new or maybe lift weights to build muscle and bone.

EXAMPLES:

"I feel my muscles growing stronger as I enjoy lifting more and more."

"I celebrate my body with weekly yoga."

"My exercise routine gets me going each day and I feel stronger and stronger."

2) Write this one about your food.

EXAMPLES:

"I can be satisfied with three small meals a day."

"Getting all my photos sorted is my evening activity." (Instead of snacking.)

"I love raw vegetables and protein because I'm satisfied when I eat them."

3) Write this one about your attitude toward food. It's time to stop being at war with food. It's time to make peace with eating. Food is fuel. It isn't love, acceptance, a shield to hide behind, or a way to avoid feelings.

EXAMPLES:

"Nothing tastes as good as slim feels."

"My family and friends love me, not my food."

"I am proud that I stay on my Plan no matter where I eat." *Write below, three positive statements about your weight release outcome.*

2) Create Your Own Goals

No one but you can create your own future. You are in charge and in control. Make your goals centered on your behaviors, habits, and feelings. You can't control what others do, you can only control yourself.

I want you to write out 3 goals you want to achieve with your weight. They cannot depend on someone else. Believe me, I've heard a lot of excuses and I've made my own excuses. So, don't tell me you can't eat healthy because your family won't eat that way. It's not OK to say that you can't eat healthy because you spend too much time on the road or taking kids to practice or working long hours. And don't tell me you just don't like certain foods so you can't eat healthy.

You must decide right now that you will eat healthy because you deserve to give your body the best fuel ever. Your body needs to live and work and play hard but it needs good fuel to do it.

Just think about your car. You depend on your car to get you to your job and everywhere else you need to be. You wouldn't pour a bag of sugar into your gas tank! No! Because your car's engine would gum up and wouldn't be able to run on sugar.

But the most delicate engine in the world is the human body. It tries hard to function well on the fuel you give it and the other maintenance it needs. It needs sleep, it needs movement and it needs high-quality food. But it can't go on forever with low-quality food, sleep or little exercise. If you keep that up, your body how will start to give out.

So, when writing your goals, avoid the behavior of others such as, *"My spouse has to eat the same meals as I."* Or, *"I stay on my* eating program when my family will eat that way." Or, "I eat healthy unless we have practice or a birthday or a holiday."

In Your Notebook:

Write 3 goals here centered on your feelings and behavior.

1) Write this about how you plan to feel about holiday and special occasion meals. These are no longer eating plan busters. You've done that all of your life. Now, we look at these stressful days when we allowed food to be pushed on us or gave in to base desires about food as just another day on our program. Special occasions are about the people and memories, they are not about reinforcing unhealthy foods or eating habits.

EXAMPLES:

"Holiday and special occasion eating are so easy and stress-free because I stay on my eating plan. I enjoy the people and leave the food as fuel."

"I eat at home before holiday meals. It makes staying on my eating plan so easy."

"I can enjoy my planned food no matter who I eat with or what day it is."

2) Write this one about your behaviors around food. You may take a stressful day or emergency or boredom as excuses to eat poorly and go off your eating plan. You will stay on that Ferris Wheel of Fear if you continue: yo-yoing your way up and down the scale but never staying at a slim weight and never feeling good about yourself. It's time to stop that behavior.

EXAMPLES:

"I love eating healthy and nutritious foods daily."

"It feels good to plan out my meals a week in advance. I only think about food once."

"I have emergency eating plans, just in case. I know how to stay on my eating plan in any situation."

3) Write this one about your everyday feelings and behaviors with food. Maybe when you get home tired from your day, you feel you "deserve" to eat foods not on your plan. It's a reward for getting through the day. No doubt you deserve a reward but it DOES NOT have to be food. Reward yourself in another way. You could call and talk to a friend, you could work on sorting family pictures, maybe you could make a really cool picture book of recipes from your family with the picture of the author and a little story about her, there are all kinds of rewards you can give yourself that are not food.

EXAMPLES:

"In the evening I enjoy taking time to write that book I've always dreamed of."

"Afternoons are when I feel good about eating a high-protein snack that clears my brain."

"I drive a new way home that takes me through a neighborhood with pretty houses and I like how that feels." (Instead of by all the restaurants that tempt me.)

3) Swiss Cheese Your Motivation

How do you eat an elephant? One bite at a time!

If your goal seems huge and daunting, then it's too big. Swiss cheese it! Take out little holes one at a time and before you know it, you've hit a milestone.

So, set yourself an attainable goal that adds up to a bigger goal down the road.

Instead of thinking, "Two pounds a week will not be enough. I'll still be fat!", try thinking this way, "Losing two pounds a week is the safe and steady way to go. At that rate, I'll be twenty-four pounds slimmer in three months. Won't I look good in some new clothes?!"

In your Notebook:

Write out one Swiss Cheese Goal:

EXAMPLES:

"When I achieve a 5-pound goal, then I can change my perspective to another 5 pounds. I look at my plan in 5-pound chunks. That is so easy to attain!"

"I'm getting through each day one at a time. Each and every day gets easier and easier."

"I stick to my eating plan each and every day. My goal is to stick to my eating plan and the rest will come."

4) Calculate Your Future Weight for an Upcoming Event

Now that you've defined your goal, it's time to give your mind a treat. A little glimpse of the future that will motivate your mind to support you on your way.

Think of an event a few weeks out from now. It could be a party, a class reunion or maybe just the start of the golf season but choose an event and figure your weight loss for that day.

Here's how to do it:

Most people average a 5-pound loss the first week on this program. After that most lose one to two pounds per week. So, if your event is six weeks from now, you would calculate your loss like this:

Week 1 = 5 pounds lost

Week 2 = 2 pounds lost

Week 3 = 2 pounds lost

Week 4 = 2 pounds lost

Week 5 = 2 pounds lost

Week 6 = 2 pounds lost

   15 pounds total lost

You can estimate losing fifteen pounds over the next six weeks.

Now, go out this week and buy a new piece of clothing that will fit you when you have released fifteen pounds. This piece of clothing is a Vision Board for your subconscious mind. Hang it in a spot where you'll see it each morning and each evening before sleep.

It's important that it's new. It needn't be expensive. It can be a tee shirt or a belt; a blouse or a pair of shorts. But, make it something new for you to fit in at the time of your event.

Do NOT pick an item you already own from your closet.

In Your Notebook:

Write down a future event that is special to you. This can be a holiday, a vacation, a birthday, a class reunion, the start of summer when you plant your garden or any other time that you know you would like to look slimmer and trimmer. Now, calculate the number of weeks away this goal day falls. Estimate your weight loss weekly for this time. If you have trouble moving the scales, you can change your weekly goal to 1 pound per week. Some medical conditions or medication you take may affect this. You and your doctor can decide this together.

Once you have the number of pounds you have projected to lose, buy that new piece of clothing! It's so exciting!

5) Picture Yourself at Your Goal Weight

Now and in the future I want you to picture yourself at your goal weight. I had a hard time with this myself. But I learned there are a couple of ways to do it.

You can picture yourself at a younger age when you looked slimmer. Pull out an old picture of yourself and tape it into your notebook or out where you can see it. Keep that body in your mind and allow your mind to pull you to it like a magnet!

Another way to accomplish picturing your slimmer self is to find an image of someone you consider to have the size you desire and print out their picture. Try to make it someone of similar height and body type. Now, take a picture of you and cut your face out to tape on the body in the picture! It might sound funny but your Subconscious Mind doesn't know the difference between real and imagined. It will take that picture into your brain as reality and will pull you toward that image.

In Your Notebook:

Glue that picture of a slim and trim you into your notebook and look at it repeatedly. We're getting your Subconscious Mind accustomed to seeing you this way so you will feel comfortable in your skin. Many people lose weight but reject the smaller size in the deep part of their mind because it doesn't feel "right" or "normal."

---

6) Week One Homework

A) Weight Yourself

Post your start weight in your notebook.

(Only weigh yourself once per week.)

B) Take Body Measurements

Take your measurements and note them in your notebook.

(Measure yourself once per month.)

Here is a diagram showing where to take your measurements.

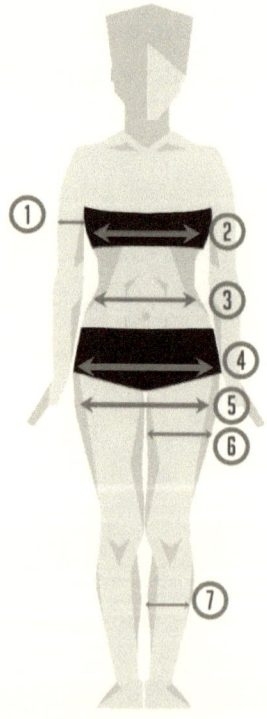

C)   Learn   Tapping   on   my   Website, www.IndianaHypnosisCenter.com, so you can use the bonus HypnoMeditation recordings each week.

D) Listen to Session One, Weight Loss Epiphany, twice a day (before dinner is a good time).

E) Tap along to your *HypnoMeditation for Weight Loss* once a day.

This week's affirmation: *I will vent out what is holding me back from losing weight, in early morning dreams.*

Week Two

Welcome to Week Two! You've made it through your first seven days of Weight Loss Epiphany! Aren't you surprised how easy it was? You can be so proud of yourself for what you've accomplished.

It's time to weight in again and you can post your current weight in your notebook. Put Week One's weight and then post today's weight and calculate the difference. Congratulations!

Wow, you are doing so well and I'm proud of you for making it to this point.

This week we'll be setting new goals to help you along the way and creating a challenge, as well. I want to see if you're up to it. You know you are.

We'll be covering these points:

- Walking challenge.

- Read the Four Key Ingredients to Weight Loss Success

- Show off and hang your new piece of clothing.

- Explain Slim and Fit Thinking vs. Fat Thinking

- Receive your Week Two homework assignment.

1) The Walking Challenge

This week I'd like to challenge you to walk 10,000 steps daily. This is an easy way to kick start your fitness. You probably already walk in your everyday life at home and at work. But now you'll be able to see just how much you do and challenge yourself to do more.

To give you an idea of how 10,000 steps balance out, 2000 steps is about one mile. And in 1/2 hour, the average person walks about 3000 steps. So, when you put in 10,000 steps, you are putting in about a five-mile walk.

Now, you could be in a situation where walking five miles is not up to your current physical ability. I recommend that you touch base with your doctor about your fitness level.

You can use an alternative workout in this case; like Tai Chi, swimming, Yoga or isometric exercises and stretching. The idea is to get moving in *some way*.

For most of you, walking is a good exercise. I suggest you download a free App on your phone to measure your walking. Go to the App Store you prefer and type in "pedometer." You will see a selection. Choose the one that most appeals to you.

In Your Notebook:

Post the number of steps you've walked each day this week.

It can be really fun to use different colors for days when you hit your goal or give yourself stickers for doing well. I like stickers and colors. That makes the posting more fun for me.

2) The Four Keys to Weight Loss Success

A) *Truthfulness*

At this turning point in your life, it's time to look closely at yourself and face the music. How do I feel about where I am? How did I get here? It might be time to admit your own responsibility for your situation. Look at yourself and take charge of your life. Ask yourself why do you do the things you do?

B) *Responsibility*

It's time to look in the mirror and think about where you are. Now take on the responsibility to make a change. It's your job to change your habits no matter what has happened in your life. This is not about assigning blame. It's about recognizing that YOU have control, to show you're willing to take charge and make changes, a little at a time. And to move yourself into a better place; mentally, physically and spiritually.

C) *Commitment*

Take that commitment you already have toward your family, pets, children, job, friends, and causes and add yourself into that same category. It's time to make yourself just as important as your kids, your relationship and your job! Pledge to yourself and take it seriously. You are worthy of your care and you deserve it. Take your life back!

D) *Inner Strength*

You're going to face challenges but, even though it might not be easy, you will get through with inner strength, understanding, and determination. You will need the patience to learn to understand and empathize with yourself. But overcoming each challenge increases that self-esteem and motivation. Once you overcome one hurdle, the next one is a little easier. Hypnosis can and will increase this inner strength and motivation from within. Each step on this journey makes you stronger and more determined in your goal; a healthier, happier life.

You deserve to love yourself enough to improve your health.

3) Show off and hang your new piece of clothing

By now you've purchased your new piece of clothing. I'd love to hear about it and see a picture! Go to our Facebook group and share with us!

Now hang your clothing in a spot where you will see it when falling asleep and waking in the morning. This is the Golden Half Hour. That time when you are naturally in hypnosis. Since your Subconscious Mind is open at this time, it will look at this piece of clothing, recognize its purpose and work hard to draw you to it. That means your subconscious mind "sees" your purpose of releasing weight and steps up to the plate; helping you make your way into that clothing!

With your new clothing, hang a copy of that image of your slimmer self you created this week. Draw your Subconscious Mind to the new you and the new clothing. Isn't this exciting?

4) Slim and Fit Thinking vs. Fat Thinking

Did you ever wonder why some people seem to go through life, facing food easily and keeping their size with little effort? At the same time, some of us struggle with our size and worry over what we eat; making each bite seemingly "bad" or "good."

That's because some people have *Slim and Fit Thinking* and others have Fat Thinking. Let me explain.

Slim and Fit Thinking people do not soothe their emotions with food. Fat Thinking people eat when they're anxious, sad, upset and even when they're happy and celebrating. *Slim and Fit Thinkers might even stop eating when their emotions are high. They might say, "I'm just too upset to eat!" Slim and Fit Thinkers find other ways to handle stress like talking it out with a friend, soaking in a bubble bath or going for a run. They might prefer to take action like looking up information and formulating a plan.* Fat Thinkers use food to distract themselves from the upset. The upset is still there but, for a little while, they are eating it away. The problem is that later, Fat Thinkers regret the eating and are disappointed in themselves thus compounding the problem.

Overweight persons can be drawn to food through external cues like ads on TV, pictures of food on social media, seeing another person eating, smelling food or thinking of a person who used to cook for them. *Slim and Fit people eat from internal cues. They might notice a feeling in their stomach, they might be yawning or feel fuzzy, or their mouth might be wanting that certain flavor. They might even drink a full glass of water before indulging, just to see if they were thirsty and not hungry.*

Fat Thinking people eat until ... they might eat until their plate is clean, eat very quickly, eat past the time when they feel satisfied, wolf down their food while absorbed in TV or the computer or their phone. *Slim and Fit Thinking people will pause after every few bites and take stock. When they feel satisfied, they stop eating, no matter how good it tastes. They just reject that hard stomach feeling that overeating makes.*

Fat Thinking people attach emotion to their food. "This cookie is calling my name." "Chocolate is my downfall." "I can't resist potato chips." "I need my comfort food." *But to Slim and Fit Thinkers, this is ridiculous. To them, food is just something you use when hungry, otherwise, no big deal. Even when the food is tasty, Slim and Fit Thinkers can be satisfied with a taste or a couple of bites.* **After all, it's the first two bites of any food that tastes the best, right?**

Fat Thinkers use denial when their weight creeps up. They often stay away from the scale because seeing the numbers brings them down. This can really send your weight out of control. *Slim and Fit Thinkers use the scales as a tool. When their weight fluctuates over two to three pounds, they make changes right away to bring it in line.*

In Your Notebook:

Write one statement you say when feeling a craving.

EXAMPLES:

"That chocolate is calling my name."

"Beer is my friend."

"I have to have pizza."

Now, write down the opposite of the statement you wrote above.

EXAMPLES:

"That chocolate is calling my name." Write a truer statement. "Chocolate is taking up too much room in my head. What I really need is to have more protein with my meal so my blood sugar doesn't influence my thinking."

"Beer is my friend." Write a truer statement. A friend doesn't make you fat or make you overeat. Beer is just something I crave when I really need to stretch and relax from stress for a few minutes.

"I have to have pizza." Write a truer statement. I have had enough pizza in my life to feed a village! I don't have to have it. I can be satisfied with healthier foods. I can research alternate ways to make pizza a healthier alternative. No one and nobody make me do anything.

5) Week Two Homework

A) Weigh Yourself

Post your weight in your notebook and subtract to find your total weight loss.

B) Listen to Session Two, Finding Satisfaction, at least once a day.

C) Listen to your HypnoMeditation for Safety in Weight Loss, once a day.

D) Use your Slim and Trim Thinking.

This week's affirmation:

I release old ideas about good and respect all my body does for me.

Week Three

Welcome to Week Three! By now you're hitting your stride and are feeling pretty great about yourself! You can be proud of your progress and I'll bet the realization is coming to you that this is the easiest program you've ever been on. Won't it be easy to continue through your life eating three small meals a day?

It's time to weight in again and you can post your current weight in your notebook. Put Week Two's weight and then post today's weight and calculate the difference. Congratulations!

You are a star! This is getting easier and easier. As you reinforce these new eating behaviors day by day, the new ways become just a way of life. You're the type of person who takes on new behavior quickly and completely. People are noticing something new about you.

This week, we're meeting new challenges with a one-two punch!

We'll be covering these points:

- Re-cap your walking challenge
- Write a self-image paragraph
- Learn Self Hypnosis

1) Re-cap Your Walking Challenge

Your challenge was to work on walking 10,000 steps per day using a pedometer or a pedometer app or an alternative exercise.

In your Notebook:

List the time limit of your workout or the number of times you fulfilled your goal. It's all good!

EXAMPLES:

"I met my goal of 10,000 steps 4 days last week."

"I did stretches 6 mornings and 3 yoga workouts last week."

"I went to the batting cage once, walked a mile 3 times and road a stationary bike 3 days for 20 minutes last week."

Now, list how you measured up to the physical challenge this week and how *you* plan to move your body this coming week. *EXAMPLES:*

"This week I will meet my goal of 10,000 steps 6 days."

"This week I plan to work out at my gym 3 times for 30 minutes, swim 2 times for 20 minutes, and walk at the mall once for 30 minutes."

"This week I'm playing racquetball once, going out in my kayak 3 times for 30 minutes and riding my bike for 3 miles."

2) Write a Self Image Paragraph

This is a description of who you are, but you're not writing about the Present Moment You, you are writing about the Future You who is Slim and Fit.

In Your Notebook:

What we will do here is write about the Future You but say it in the present tense as if it has already happened.

Let me show you what I mean. Your Future Self will be as a Slim and Fit person; a big change from the person you started as when we began Weight Loss Epiphany. So, the Future You might be described as something like this in your mind:

"I will wear size ten clothing. I will look in the mirror then and like what I see. My son will hug me and say, "I can reach all the way around you now!" I will go on rides at Disneyland and fit in all the seats. People won't look at me that way they do now. I will be proud of myself and not need all the medications I do now."

But we want the Subconscious Mind to buy into our new image and want to take us there. To do that, we must take out words like "will" and "won't." When you use future tense words like those, the Subconscious Mind blows you off. It doesn't believe in some make-believe future. You've been telling it for years you would go on a diet Monday morning! The Subconscious Mind only believes in the NOW and is only motivated by NOW. So, let's go back and re-write that self-image paragraph in the NOW!

"I comfortably wear size ten clothing. When I look in the mirror, I like what I see. My son is hugging me, saying, "I can reach all the way around you now!" I am riding at Disneyland on any ride I want and I fit beautifully in any seat. I love how I look and how others admire my fitness. I am so proud of myself. My doctor says I don't need all of those medications anymore!"

Write your Self-Image Paragraph.

3) Learn Self-Hypnosis

Self-hypnosis is easy and practical. You can learn it here but the lesson will last you a lifetime. You need not use it more than a few minutes a day but the change you can make in your life can be profound.

Here is how you do it in a few easy steps:

a) In your notebook: plan out the issue and then follow the steps to the solution

Spell out the problem you wish to address, then plan it in your notebook. (Use the enclosed examples as your guide.)

b) Slip into hypnosis. You've been practicing with the recorded sessions and now you can do it on your own. There are many ways, such as focusing on a spot on the wall, counting yourself down from five to zero (deep sleep) or flexing and relaxing your muscle groups one at a time. Come into that state of focused attention.

c) Focus on the solution to your problem thinking over how you will think, feel and act.

d) Imagine, picture or pretend you are carrying out the new behavior. This is called a Mental Rehearsal.

e) State positive affirmations so you can remind yourself about creating this change you want.

f) Now, craft your own post-hypnotic suggestion like this:

From now on, when I encounter (this) _____, I (do this) _____.

g) Come up and out: open your eyes, count yourself up from zero to five and give a big stretch.

That's all there is to it! I've made an example to start you and it uses a strong commitment to change. Your commitment to change should look like this:

- Focused on the positive

- Using your own strengths

- Contains statements that rely on what you think, what you feel, and what you say and what you do

- All about the solution, not problem-based

- Always based in the future

- Focused on your own actions, not depending on anyone else or something outside of you to happen

- Specific. This solution should occur at a certain time and place where you implement your solution. When (this) happens, I (do this). Stay away from vague thinking like, I want to be happier.

- Use all your senses. Your words and what you visualize, even what you smell, have big effects on your Subconscious Mind.

You can plan your session following the example and then you can go into self-hypnosis as I described. Or you can record your own voice reading out the hypnosis session to use later. You might prefer having the recording to just listen to and concentrate on. Here, you plan your session in your notebook, then use your device or phone to record your self-hypnosis session. Have fun with it and use all the wording and positive reinforcement you can.

In Your Notebook:

EXAMPLE:

Sample Self-Hypnosis One by Judith Pearson, PhD

- *Describe your problem or concern.*

  I eat whenever I feel stressed out like when someone criticizes me.

- *Self-hypnosis induction. Take three deep breaths and count yourself down.*

- *Create the solution: what is your new response? How will you think, act and feel?*

  New thinking: *Criticism is only another person's opinion. It is not necessarily accurate. I can treat it just like information that may or may not be useful.*

  New feeling: *I detach from the criticism so I can remain objective about it.*

  New actions: *I respond calmly and tactfully.*

- *Visualize yourself carrying out this new action in a situation that previously would have been challenging. This is your mental rehearsal.*

I visualize a co-worker criticizing one of my reports, saying things I feel are unfair. I take a deep breath and feel relaxed. I tell myself that the criticism is only information for me to evaluate. I feel calm and detached. I calmly look at the co-worker and say, "I'll gladly listen to any specific recommendations for improvement."

- *Your positive affirmations.*

The calmer I feel, the more I make wise choices about food. I am in charge of my own self-esteem, and no one else can take it away from me. I eat only when I feel hungry. When I feel stressed, I seek solutions, not more food!

- *Your post-hypnotic suggestion:*

From now on, whenever I encounter someone criticizing me, I calmly take a deep breath and recall that I am in charge of my self-esteem and feelings. I think clearly and remind myself that I am okay and criticism is only information. I respond *calmly and tactfully. I feel good about it afterward.*

- *Bring yourself up and out. Count up from zero to five, give a big stretch and take a deep breath. You're done!*

In Your Notebook:

Now you know the steps, write out what you want to accomplish and practice Self-Hypnosis.

4) Week Three Homework

A) Weigh Yourself

Post your new weight in your notebook and subtract to find your total weight loss.

B) Listen to Session Three Recording, "New Path", at least once a day.

C) Listen and participate in your HypnoMeditation, "Tapping for Clarity" once a day.

D) Write out a solution to a problem following your Self-Hypnosis guidelines and use self-hypnosis to implement your plan.

This Week's Affirmation:

My confidence rises each day and encouragement seems to appear in my mind as if I were my own best friend.

Week Four

Congratulations, you've made it to Week Four, into Success! You have successfully made this way of eating a habit that can take you into a new vision for the rest of your life. You may have been struggling for a long time with your weight or it might be something that cropped up as new to you after having a baby or changing jobs or a trauma that happened. No matter what caused you to gain weight, now you know how to release it. You don't even have to struggle like so many do. You don't have to give up lists of your favorite foods. It's just that easy.

Now it's time to finish this part of your journey of discovery. You aren't done. You've only just begun. This is how to eat from here on out. Even though you won't have more workbook chapters to work on, this is not the end of your insights into your own self-motivation. Using the recordings daily to reinforce the habit, using self-hypnosis to overcome bumps in the road, and changing your self-talk to present tense and positive affirmations, is how to make all the rest of the changes you make in your life. It's the way to keep this way of eating and thinking a permanent habit.

You can be proud of yourself! You've made huge strides! It isn't all about the scales either. Changing your habits around food is very hard and you've done it! You've impressed yourself by doing something impressive!

In this fourth assignment, you will:

- Learn the Four R's and put them into practice.

- File a Personal Injury Suit against Perfectionism

- Write a Thank You Note

- Have a Talk from Your Old Self

- Receive your last homework assignment

1) Learn the Four R's

It's time to put a stop to all the negative self-talk that you say to yourself all day long. It's like a tape that runs on a loop in your head all day long. And, boy, are we mean to ourselves! We've practiced talking to ourselves in the present tense and eliminating negatives. Now, let's get down to the nitty-gritty and blast that mean stuff completely out of our head.

- *Reframing*

Maybe you say things to yourself that are mean but you think you need to be mean or you will never reform. Has that really helped you make meaningful changes so far? You need not cut yourself down to discipline yourself. Maybe the intent behind the words is positive. So, let's just rephrase it so it is inspiring rather than intimidating. Because, I don't know about you, but I rebel against anything that tries to intimidate me.

Like this: you might think, "I'm too dumb to learn to dance (swim, Pilates, yoga, Tai Chi or whatever) for exercise." The intent behind this is positive, you want to exercise in a new way but you don't want to look foolish. So, we reframe the wording so it is positive and supportive. " I find new ways to exercise that are fun. I learn these new ways with other beginners so we are all in the same stage of learning." You might feel more confident if you come into something new with a little practice. "I find new ways to exercise that are fun and I take a few lessons on YouTube first to get the hang of it."

In Your Notebook:

Rewrite one of the old messages you play in your head and reframe it to the positive.

EXAMPLES:

"I can never lose weight because being fat runs in my family." <u>Reframe and write a truer statement.</u> "Most of my family is overweight but fat is not hereditary. My family's metabolism runs very efficiently and that's how our bloodline stayed alive through famine. I celebrate my superior body! I release weight and keep it off with this new way of eating and moving for the rest of my life."

"I have a bad knee so I can't exercise enough to be strong." <u>Reframe and write a truer statement.</u> "My knee is not able to do some workouts so I find new ways to work out that don't strain my knee, just like people who have lost their legs can work out from a wheelchair or a special seated ski."

"I can't eat this way forever! I'm just going to diet for a month." <u>Reframe and write a truer statement.</u> "I eat the Weight Loss Epiphany way forever. I can eat anything but I only eat 3 small meals a day and am satisfied after a few bites."

- *Refuting*

When you say something silly and just mean to yourself, convince yourself that it isn't true. Give yourself evidence and don't take the criticism. For example, you might say to yourself, "I'll never meet my goal. It's too hard." Don't take that kind of talk! Remember just what's on the line your self-worth.

Refute it with evidence: "I don't believe any statement that says 'never' because that's just an exaggeration. I've faced many hard things in my life and I came through those. I can do this, too. It's not even close to as hard as those times were. I'm a lot tougher than I seem."

In Your Notebook:

Refute something you always seem to tell yourself.

EXAMPLES:

"I just love to eat! I just love food! How can I ever reach my goal and keep going?" Refute and write a truer statement. "Of course, I love food and eating, everyone does. I'm not special in that regard. Every day I'm closer to my goal. Every day this way of eating gets easier and easier. I remember when learning to drive was hard on the first day, but every day it became easier and easier."

"Nobody eats this way. My family will hate me if I don't eat like them on holidays and birthdays." Refute and write a truer statement. "I have a small amount of whatever I choose on holidays and birthdays, I'm not deprived. What my family wants for me is great health. They stand with me and my healthy way of life."

"If I eat this way forever, I might have terrible cravings every day and then I'll just go off it like every other diet I've tried." Refute and write a truer statement. "If I eat this way forever, I will never have a weight problem again. I eat this way forever because I love life and want to increase my joy. Weight Loss Epiphany isn't a diet. Diets aren't sustainable, that's why I always fail at them. Weight Loss Epiphany is sustainable and easy. I love to eat this way every day."

- *Refusal*

Don't allow yourself to listen to the negatives. When you hear a put-down in your head, whether it's your voice or someone else's, just stop and say to yourself," No! I refuse to listen to this stuff. I don't deserve it and I would never talk like this to my child or even my pet! I certainly won't take it from my own self!"

Imagine that your mind is like a television. If you don't like a show, you change the channel. So, if you hear the crappy talk, change the channel!

In Your Notebook:

Write a negative you seem to tell yourself often. Then write out the refusal.

EXAMPLES:

"You're such a stupid dummy." <u>Refuse and write a truer statement.</u> "I am neither stupid nor dumb. I'm an intelligent person that sometimes jumps in without thinking but I have a good heart. I'm going to stop and pause the next time something comes up so that I make the best choice for me. I've made other smart choices, I can do it again."

"You're fat and you'll always be a fat slob." <u>Refuse and write a truer statement.</u> "I don't curse that way to myself any longer. I don't allow that kind of put down from others and I won't take it from myself. I am healthier each week as I eat well and stay on my plan. I am doing what I need to do for myself and family and that means staying on my plan. I love staying on my plan because it means I don't have to think about food."

"You've never stayed this long on a diet. You're going to fail. You want to fail." <u>Refuse and write a truer statement.</u> "I want to succeed and releasing weight has never been this simple. I am succeeding and every day I find it easier and easier."

- *Replacement*

Consciously stop yourself and replace the negative talk with a positive right away! It's hard at first but in a very short time, you'll find yourself doing it on autopilot.

So many of us find it hard to say, "I love and accept myself, respecting my body and my mind." But we have no problem thinking, "I'll always be fat and I just can't change that." This is Stuck Thinking and it leads to unhealthy patterns of behavior. Your subconscious is listening and it will carry out your negative orders. So, order up some of the good life instead!

In Your Notebook:

Write out a phrase or sentence you say to yourself that's rude and mean. Then, write out its opposite.

EXAMPLES:

"You'll never amount to anything." <u>Replace and write a true statement.</u> "I achieve everything I dream to do. I use effort and hard work with determination to reach any goal."

"Who would ever look at you? You're no fashion model." <u>Replace and write a true statement.</u> "Beauty shines out from the inside of a person and I shine my beauty each day. I'm lit with a lovely light from within. That's what people see in me to love. I am loved and I love."

2) A Personal Injury Suit against Perfectionism

Are you tough on yourself, always holding yourself to a standard higher than anyone else? At the end of the day, do you always think about all the things you didn't do? You're might be a perfectionist.

Trying to always be perfect is a standard none of us can live up to. If you think you have to be perfect, you'll be disappointed every day of your life. I think you should sue yourself for pain and suffering damages! It's terrible to live each day feeling you're not good enough and never measuring up to your own imagination.

Eating is no way to escape self-criticism. I suggest that instead of trying to be perfect and failing each day, you should shoot for Excellence. Isn't Excellence an awesome standard to live by? And Excellence is attainable and a worthy goal to achieve for anyone. You have a margin of error with Excellence we need as humans.

In Your Notebook:

List a couple of ways you can allow yourself to be human and Excellent.

EXAMPLES:

"The undone at the end of my list today is the beginning of my list for tomorrow. My tombstone will not say, "She didn't finish her list."

"I have made poor choices in my life but when I learned better, I strove to do better."

"I meet my physical body where it is. Some days it wants to do more and eat more and some days it wants to do less and eat less."

3) A Thank You Note

It's high time you wrote a thank you note to your body. It might not be perfect or look the way you want it to yet. It might feel like sometimes the two of you are in a battle. But that's not true. Your Subconscious Mind directs your body to protect you at all costs and it takes the information you feed it to do this. It uses all of your senses; sight, smell, touch, taste, and hearing, to take in messages and allow your body to react accordingly. It also considers your memories and self-talk as a guide in how to behave and protect yourself.

For the whole of your life, your body has done its best to heal you when you're hurt, to pump in strength when you're threatened, to alert you when it needs maintenance and to save up for hard times. And how do you show your gratitude? Well, using this program, Weight Loss Epiphany, is one way to reward your body and mind with positive improvement in your thoughts and actions. But let's give credit where credit is due. Even though you've done your darndest to overlook the messages from your body about what it needs like "I'm full, I need to move more, I need more rest and sleep, I can't function on alcohol alone," your body still found ways to recover and keep you going. So, let's acknowledge all your body does for you and promise to listen to the signals your body gives you a little better.

In Your Notebook:

Write a thank you note to your physical body and acknowledge all that it's done for you. Make your promise to it to be faithful to what it's asking for, never to ignore its signals to you and support its health the way it supports you.

EXAMPLES:

"Dear Body,

I want to thank you for all you've done for me during this life of mine. You've held me up with strong legs when I needed to get through my workday. You've realized that there could be lean times with little food so you saved in fat cells energy to use just in case. Even though I've eaten poor nutritional foods, you took all the nutrition you could and kept me going. I thank you.

My promise to you is to stop ignoring your signals to me. Stop eating when I'm satisfied, move more when you're stiff and achy from sitting too long and understand that high-quality fuel is what you truly need.

I love you,

Me XOXO"

"Dear Body,

Thank you for how you've carried me through all my years of abusing you. I'm very sorry about that. You've stood by me throughout all of these times when I didn't pay attention to you. Even when you tried to show me you were undernourished in vitamins and high-quality food, I just ignored that and ate what I wanted, when I wanted it.

Through it all you've been good to me, getting me to school and work and taking care of my family. I can't believe you put up with my abuse all this time. Thanks for not bringing me down with a heart attack or stroke even though I may have deserved it. I promise you that I'm ready to listen to your signals and give you fuel that you can really use. It's time to pay you back for all of your goodness to me.

XOXO,

Me"

4) A Talk From Your Old Self

This is the place where we write a note to our Future Self who is slim and fit. Write to that person who will look at this a year from now. Give your future self some advice about continuing this healthy lifestyle you've begun.

In Your Notebook:

Write a note to your Future Self from the viewpoint of today. Tell yourself what you feel like now and encourage the Future You to never return to the bad habits you had until now.

EXAMPLES:

Dear Self,

Here I sit today, overweight and miserable, hoping and wanting this to be the last time I'm ever at this weight in my life. I have to have a bunch of medications just to keep me alive. My clothes are feeling tight again. I hate the way I look and the way people look at me. I feel like a failure.

Actually, scratch all that. For the last few weeks that I've been using Weight Loss Epiphany, I've shown myself that I can change the way I eat and feel. I can move more and be stronger. I have the key to eating for the rest of my life. I want to commit to that way. So when you're reading this again and a year from now. I want to see that you've kept that commitment and you're feeling more fit and slim than you have in a long, long time.

I want to know that you have been able to feel and look great. I want to hear from the doctor that we don't need all that medication anymore. I want you to look around and know that people admire what you've done and wish they could do it, too. I want you to NEVER be where I am today. EVER.

Let's live a long life.

I love you,

Me XOXO

5) Your last homework assignment

a) Weigh yourself.

Post your new weight in your notebook and subtract to find your total weight loss.

b) Take your monthly body measurements.

Post your new measurements and subtract from your old measurements.

How many inches have you released?

c) Listen to your recording for this week and your HypnoMeditation at least once a day.

d) Practice self-hypnosis twice this week.

It has been my privilege to be your guide on this Weight Loss Epiphany journey.

I'm proud of your progress and I would like to hear from you about it!

You can contact me at www.IndianaHypnosisCenter.com or on Facebook, Angie J. Hernandez, Certified Hypnotherapist. My hope for you is a life of continued joy and a happy relationship with yourself.

For in-person sessions, call Angie J. Hernandez, C.Ht. at (574) 658-4686.

SHOP THE FULL SERIES

Get more *Weight Loss Hypnosis* books now:

Amazon

To browse all books by Angie J. Hernandez, C.Ht.,

just click here: https://amazon.com/author/angiejhernandezcht/

View All Books

https://amazon.com/author/angiejhernandezcht/

THANK YOU!

It has been my privilege to be your guide on this Weight Loss Epiphany journey.

I'm proud of your progress and I would like to hear from you about it!

You can contact me at www.IndianaHypnosisCenter.com or on Facebook, WLE Coaching Club. My hope for you is a life of continued joy and a happy relationship with yourself.

For in-person sessions, call me using (574) 658-4686.

XO,
Angie J. Hernandez, C.Ht.

For updates about current and upcoming releases, as well as exclusive promotions, visit the author's website at:

Amazon Author Page:
https://amazon.com/author/angiejhernandezcht/

Author Website:
https://indianahypnosiscenter.com/

Got a Question?

Leave a comment here:

https://www.facebook.com/groups/WLECoachingClub/

and you'll get answers!

www.ingramcontent.com/pod-product-compliance
Lightning Source LLC
Chambersburg PA
CBHW020410290526
45785CB00005B/2492